CONTENTS

Copyright © 1993 by The American National Red Cross. All rights reserved.
A Mosby Lifeline imprint of Mosby–Year Book, Inc.

RECOGNIZING

Your senses—hearing, sight, and smell—may help you recognize an emergency.

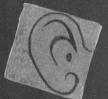

UNUSUAL NOISES
Screams, yells, moans, or calls for help
Breaking glass, crashing metal, or
    screeching tires
Changes in machinery or equipment
    noises
Sudden, loud voices

UNUSUAL SIGHTS
A stalled vehicle
An overturned pot
A spilled medicine container
Broken glass
Downed electrical wires
Smoke or fire

Emergency
Action Steps

In the excitement of an emergency, you may be frightened or confused about what to do. Stay calm, you can help. The emergency action steps will show you how.

EMERGENCIES

Emergencies are often signaled by something unusual that catches your attention.

UNUSUAL ODORS
Odors that are stronger than usual
Unrecognizable odors

UNUSUAL APPEARANCES OR BEHAVIORS
Difficulty breathing
Clutching the chest or throat
Slurred, confused, or hesitant speech
Unexplainable confusion or drowsiness
Sweating for no apparent reason
Unusual skin color

1. Check the scene and the victim.

2. Call 9-1-1 or the local emergency number.

3. Care for the victim.

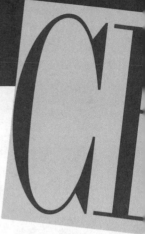

- **Check the scene for safety.**

- **Check the victim for level of consciousness, breathing, pulse, and bleeding.**

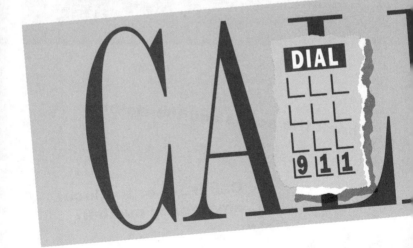

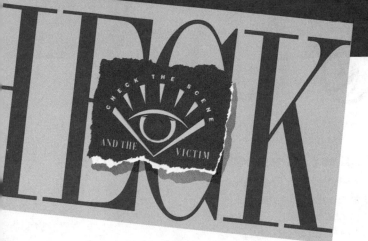

How to Call

Give the dispatcher the necessary information. Be prepared to give—

- The exact location or address of the emergency. Include nearby intersections, landmarks, and the building name, floor, or room or apartment number.
- The telephone number from which the call is being made.
- The caller's name.
- What happened.
- How many people are involved.
- The conditions of the victims.
- What help is being given.

Do not hang up until the dispatcher hangs up. The EMS dispatcher may be able to tell you how to best care for the victim until the ambulance arrives.

Return and continue to care for the victim.

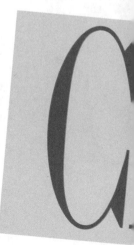

Call for an ambulance if the victim—

Is or becomes unconscious.
Has trouble breathing.
Has chest pain or pressure.
Is bleeding severely.
Has pressure or pain in the abdomen that does not
    go away.
Is vomiting or passing blood.
Has seizures, a severe headache, or slurred speech.
Appears to have been poisoned.
Has injuries to the head, neck, or back.
Has possible broken bones.

Care for life-threatening conditions first. If there are none—

- Watch for changes in the victim's
  breathing and consciousness.

- Help the victim rest comfortably.

- Keep the victim from getting chilled
  or overheated.

- Reassure the victim.

Or if the situation involves—

Fire or explosion.
Downed electrical wires.
Swiftly moving or rapidly rising water.
Presence of poisonous gas.
Vehicle collisions.
Victims who cannot be moved easily.

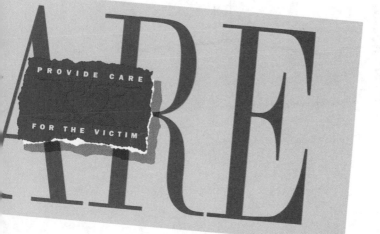

PROVIDE CARE

FOR THE VICTIM

Give abdominal thrusts

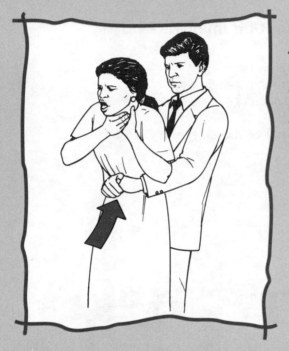

Place fist just above navel and give quick, upward thrusts until object is removed.

If Not Breathing

Give rescue breathing

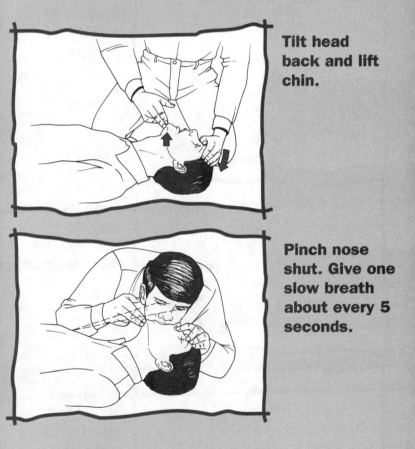

Tilt head back and lift chin.

Pinch nose shut. Give one slow breath about every 5 seconds.

If Air Won't Go In

Give abdominal thrusts

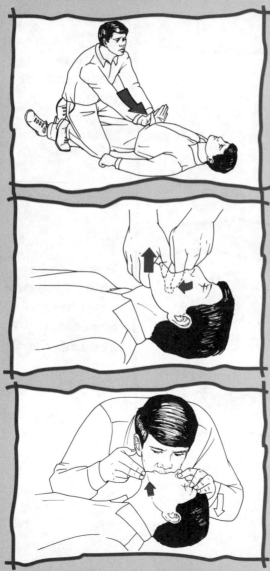

Give up to
5 abdominal
thrusts.

Look for
and clear
any objects
from mouth.

Tilt head
back and
reattempt
breaths.
Repeat steps
until breaths
go in.

Give CPR

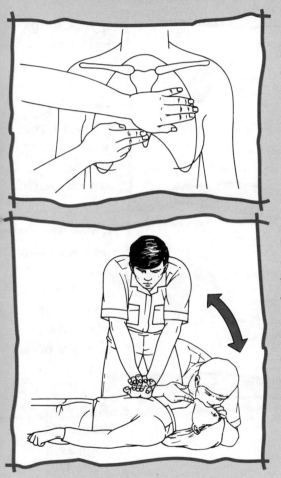

Find hand position on center of breastbone.

Compress chest 15 times. Give two slow breaths. Repeat sets of compressions and breaths until ambulance arrives.

If Bleeding

Control bleeding

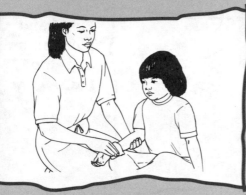

If bleeding is severe:

Apply pressure against the wound using a clean cloth.

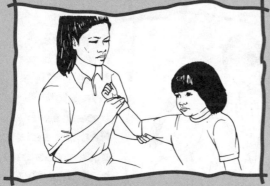

Raise the injured area if you do not think the wound involves a broken bone.

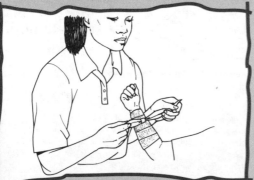

Apply a bandage snugly over the dressing.

If Burned

To care for a burn—

Stop the Burning. Put out flames or remove source.

Cool the Burn. Using large amounts of cool water.

Cover the Burn. Cover with dry, clean dressings.

If caused by—

Chemicals—— Flush skin or eyes with large amounts of cool running water.

Electricity—— Make sure power is off. Check breathing and pulse if unconscious. Cover burn with a clean, dry dressing.

A critical burn needs immediate medical attention. Call for an ambulance if a burn—

- Involves breathing difficulty.
- Covers more than one body part.
- Involves the head, neck, hands, feet, or genitals.
- Is to a child or elderly person (other than a very minor burn).
- Is caused by chemicals, explosions, or electricity.

If Unable to Move or Use Body Part

Keep the injured part from moving

Apply ice to the injury site

Get medical care

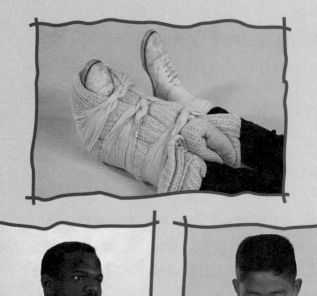

Splint—

Only if the victim must be moved.
Only if you can do it without causing more pain.
In the position you find it.

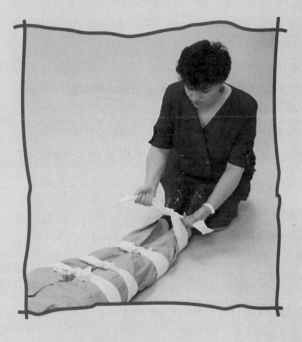

To splint an injury—

Support the injured area above and below
the site of the injury. Soft materials, such
as folded blankets, towels, pillows, folded
triangular bandages, or a triangular
bandage tied as a sling can be used.

If Suddenly Ill

Care for life-threatening conditions first. Then—

Help the victim rest comfortably.

Keep the victim from getting chilled or overheated.

Reassure the victim.

Watch for changes in consciousness and breathing.

Do not give anything to eat or drink unless the victim is fully conscious.

If the victim—

Vomits— Place the victim on his or her side.

Faints— Position victim on back and elevate legs if no head or back injury suspected.

Has a Diabetic Emergency— Give the victim some sort of sugar.

Has a Seizure— Do not hold or restrain the person or place anything between the teeth. Remove any objects that might cause injury. Cushion the victim's head using folded clothing or small pillow.

Has Been Poisoned— Call the local emergency number or the Poison Control Center.